The River Flows

Dear Mary
It was good to see you
again Hope you find this
book helpful. Christie

The River Flows

Christie E. Hoffman

Best Regards
Christie Hoffman

VANTAGE PRESS
New York

FIRST EDITION

Published by Vantage Press, Inc.
516 West 34th Street, New York, New York 10001

Manufactured in the United States of America
ISBN: 0-533-11723-2

0 9 8 7 6 5 4 3 2

To my sister, Louise Burleson

Contents

1. A New Channel Is Formed: My Life Turned into a New Direction 1
2. Like the Current in the River . . . So Was the Way of My Life 5
3. The River Changed Its Course, So Changed My Life 11
4. Like the Current of the River, Which Cleanses the River of Debris 13
5. Like Ripples on the Surface of the River, So Were the Disturbances in My Life 17
6. Like a Turbulence in the River, So My Life Seemed in a Turmoil 19
7. As the Flow of a River Nears Flood Stage, So the Problems Were Overwhelming Me 25
8. The River Seemed Like a Whirlpool as My Difficulties Increased Tremendously 31
9. Like the Gentle Flowing of the Current on Its Course in the River . . . So My Life Seemed to Flow More Peacefully 35
10. The Changing Currents of the River Were Like the Changing Events in My Life 39

Conclusion 45

The River Flows

1

A New Channel Is Formed: My Life Turned into a New Direction

Alzheimer's disease not only affects the person afflicted with the disease, but also the spouse and/or members of the family who care for the individual. The first time I realized something was wrong with my husband was on July 4, 1976, when I returned home after spending fourteen weeks in the hospital with pancreatitis.

When I arrived home, I discovered my husband had moved into the other bedroom. He said I would get "more rest" if I slept alone. I felt rejected and thought he no longer wanted me as his wife. He insisted on preparing his own meals and could not tolerate me anywhere near him when he was in the kitchen; he would immediately snatch up his food and vacate the area. He was afraid I had a contagious disease.

His work had brought him in contact with many government officials and we had attended conventions in different cities. We had both enjoyed exchanging views with the bigwigs, and conversation-wise we both had managed to hold our own. We also had enjoyed various parties at his place of work. On one occasion we had been invited on a boat ride given by one of the officials. There was dancing, which we both enjoyed

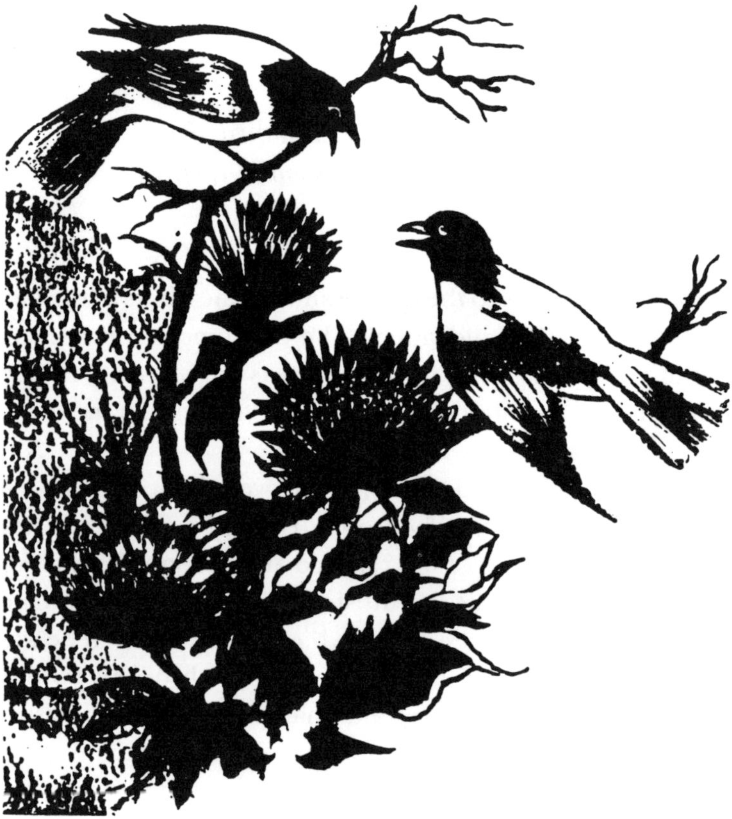

(Edmond was an excellent dancer). Those were the good days, as Edmond still enjoyed many activities.

I remember December 31, 1974, New Year's Eve. We had an open house; all his coworkers and their spouses attended. Edmond mingled with the group and he listened to some music a friend of his played on the accordion. It reminded him of when he and several friends had had a band; they had played on the radio and at dances. Now, two years later, he seemed a different person. He no longer seemed to enjoy the company of others. He would visit only with a few of his older friends and some of his relatives, but that was pretty much the extent of his socializing.

Even visits from different family members seemed to upset him. In fact, he seemed to resent their companionship. When relatives came over to visit, he would tell me they were trying to turn me against him. He was becoming more and more possessive and jealous.

By October 6, 1976, it became increasingly difficult to enjoy visits with my family. Edmond thought everyone was trying to cheat him. He even accused me of stealing his money, and there really wasn't any reasoning with him.

My husband tried to control and dominate me. He didn't think I was capable of making my own decisions, and unfortunately, because of his constant criticism, I began to lose confidence in myself, suffering loss of self-esteem. I wondered if I would ever be able to regain my sense of direction and resume my career as a nurse.

Some of my stress diminished whenever I worked in my garden or when I was outdoors close to nature. We had a bird sanctuary in the back of our garden, and when I worked in the garden, a variety of birds sang and followed me around. One day a catbird flew from tree to tree, singing and imitating other birds; the small birds enjoyed sitting on the grapevines and berry bushes as they serenaded me with their songs.

Other small birds enjoyed the company of humans as well. While I worked in the flowerbeds, they would chirp and sit on the evergreen bushes near the house; they didn't appear the least bit timid. The orioles built their nests in the cottonwood tree in our yard. It's amazing the way their nests withstand the strong winds. One day I was in the front yard standing by the apple tree. I noticed a male oriole sitting on a limb with the baby birds all lined up in a row. It appeared he was about to teach the young ones how to fly. It was a sight to behold. I was afraid to stay and watch, as I didn't want to disturb them. It was a mystery to me how they made the trip from the nest on the cottonwood tree to the limb on the apple tree.

2

Like the Current in the River . . . So Was the Way of My Life

As time passed by, Edmond seemed to be having problems at work. It was June 1977 when Edmond, upon arriving home from work, was very certain that some of his coworkers were trying to make trouble for him. Someone at work was after his job.

When things did not go his way, he became very angry and would threaten suicide with his handgun. He would say to me, "After I shoot myself dead, you will be responsible." When I discussed Edmond's suicidal threats with our family doctor, he told me I should be concerned that Edmond actually might kill himself. Our doctor suggested that my husband see a psychiatrist. Edmond refused to go, so I went alone. He kept telling me I must be crazy because I was the one going to the psychiatrist. He also accused me of having an affair with the psychiatrist, who was the same age as his grandson. I finally stopped going. The advice I received was to grow a thick skin so the criticism and negative treatment I was receiving wouldn't bother me.

My husband became very paranoid, thinking everyone was trying to cheat him. At first these symptoms would last a few days, but gradually began increasing to a week, then at

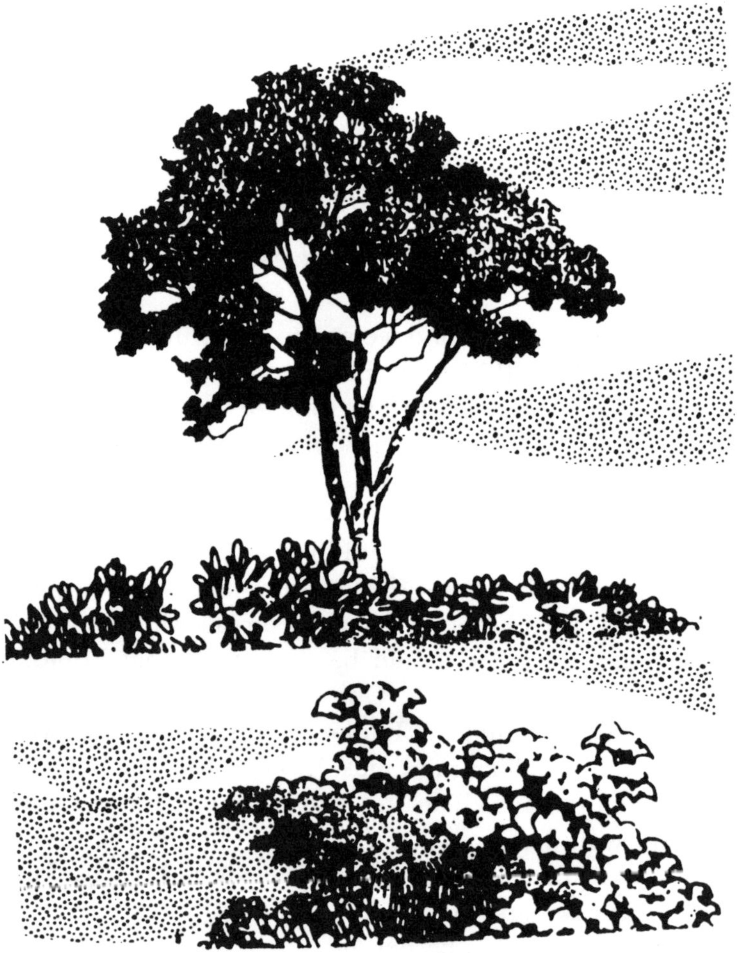

times lasting for several weeks. Again, I spoke to our family doctor, telling him I thought Edmond wasn't getting enough oxygen to his brain. The doctor ordered numerous tests to rule out blockage in the carotid artery. He made an appointment for Edmond to see a specialist. I telephoned the doctor to ask why I wasn't notified. He told me if I wanted to know anything about my husband's medical history I would have to be present when he talked to Edmond. At that time I hadn't realized the seriousness of Edmond's mental and physical condition. Edmond also had a diabetic condition and was placed on a special diet. He lost weight and became very upset; he was afraid the diet would harm him. He believed the doctor and I were trying to kill him.

In the spring of 1971, a tornado touched down and uprooted most of our trees. So in April 1977, when we built our new house, we decided to so some landscaping on our front yard. We had a garden and landscaping store deliver and plant several large trees. We also transplanted several shade trees from Edmond's brother's woods. I made up different names for the trees as I talked to them.

The trees seemed to thrive; our yard became an attractive, pleasant place in which to relax. One day, as I was walking around the yard, I noticed that our dark leaf red maple tree appeared to be dying. I had read in a book that sometimes a tree could become lazy and sometimes it was necessary for one to beat the tree with a willow switch very hard, all around the trunk, and that that would start the sap flowing. I tried the method, as I thought I had nothing to lose. I also removed the dead center. Soon the tree took on a normal look, and I was very pleased with the results.

By the summer of 1977, I seemed to be regaining my strength. My days were brightened by the antics of our two Siamese kittens, Cindy, a blue point, and Sud, a seal point. One day when I was in the yard, I noticed them coming from

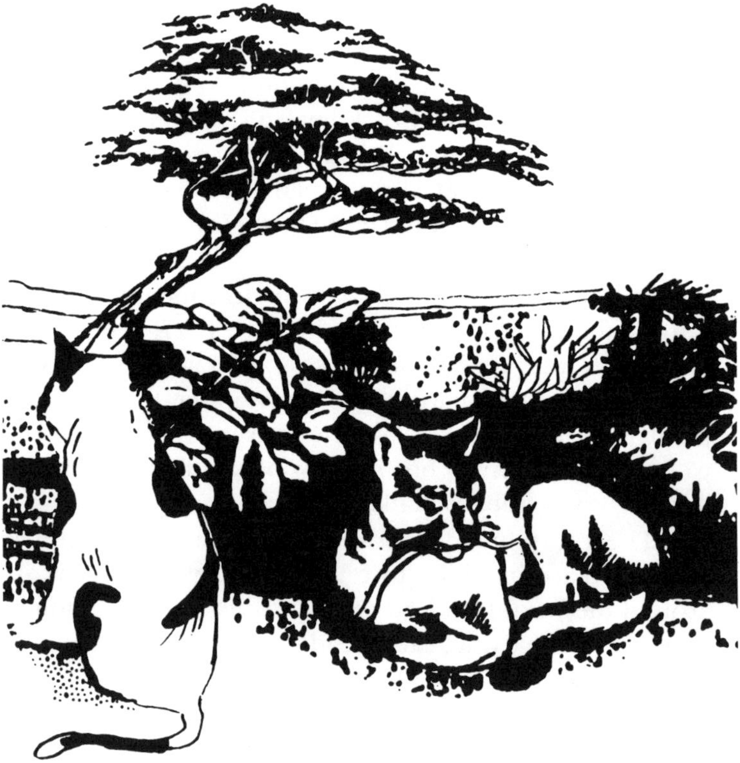

the garden area carrying something between them. Sud had the head of a grass snake in his mouth and Cindy had the tail. They dropped the snake by the front door, then looked up at me, waiting to be thanked for the gift. The expression on my face must have given them the impression I was not very grateful.

Sud was quite a talker, telling me about his various adventures as he followed me around. Cindy was also very active, jumping from tree to tree like a flying squirrel. She also liked to climb on top of doors and swing back and forth like a monkey.

In the early evenings, Edmond and I would sit outside on our porch. We enjoyed watching Sud and Cindy playing around in the yard with the young rabbits.

In the winter I spent some time feeding and watching the birds and squirrels as they came to their feeders. The cardinals always arrived early; the male cardinals with their bright red feathers made a beautiful contrast against the white snow. The smaller birds ate next, followed by the mourning doves. The last to eat were the blue jays; they were the most talkative of all.

In February 1978, while looking out the window, I noticed strong winds blowing the snow. The visibility was extremely poor and we ended up having a major snowstorm.

We were without electricity for four days. Edmond's brother was staying with us. It was a challenging time—just like in the old pioneering days. The fireplace was our only source of heat. I hung an old iron kettle over the fire to do the cooking. Edmond and I slept on a sofa bed, while his brother slept in a chair. It took a lot of time and energy to keep the fire going. The wood was stored in the garage a short distance from the house, and it was quite a problem keeping the path clear from the drifting and blowing snow.

There was no electric power for the pump, so water had

to be conserved. For washing we melted snow. Although living conditions were extremely difficult, it nevertheless was very interesting. I was glad when the electrical power was restored so I could cook on my electric stove and sleep in my bed.

The first thing we did after the storm was to purchase a bottled gas stove. Edmond's brother, Otto, continued to live with us. I enjoyed his company, especially when he told stories about family in his years of growing up. It helped me to understand Edmond better. Otto had episodes of falling down, and I always wondered why this was so; I later learned he had bone cancer.

During the following October, in 1978, Otto fell out of bed; it woke us up. I followed Edmond into Otto's bedroom. My husband was very angry at being awakened. He picked Otto up and threw him onto the bed. I was very frightened when I went back to bed. I realized if he could treat his brother this way, perhaps nothing would stop him from treating me the same way. The next morning Otto said he no longer wanted to stay with us and would like to go to the hospital. I called his doctor to make arrangements for him to be admitted. Otto stayed in the hospital for a few days before he was transferred to a nursing home.

One night I had a dream. I saw Otto and he told me he was afraid to die. I saw a hand extended out. I told Otto if he held onto the hand he would be able to cross over to a new life.

I decided to visit him the next morning. He appeared unconscious when I arrived. He didn't respond when I spoke to him, and his pulse was very weak. However, he appeared peaceful and there was a big smile on his face. On that same day, November 2, 1978, Otto died. I telephoned Edmond, his brother, and his sisters to let them know.

3

The River Changed Its Course, So Changed My Life

By June 1983, the changes apparent in my husband since our marriage had reached a critical point. I finally decided to leave and file for a divorce. I wanted to work in the hospital where I had worked prior to getting married. I drove to Ann Arbor and rented a one-bedroom apartment. I told Edmond I had filed for a divorce and was leaving, but he insisted on going with me. I consulted with my attorney; he said if we had separate bedrooms we could live in the same apartment. With little trouble, I was able to change to a two-bedroom apartment in the same complex.

Getting ready to move and having an auction sale was a major undertaking, and I seemed to have the full responsibility. I was beginning to feel exhausted and couldn't seem to get my strength back.

It was after office hours when I telephoned my doctor; I told him I was feeling dizzy and weak. I was told to go to the emergency room at the hospital. They took some tests. The EKG showed my heart was very irregular, and I was told my potassium level was very low. After several hours in the emergency room, I was admitted. At last I thought I would get some rest, but it wasn't to be. I was given potassium intravenously and frequently disturbed by members of the staff as they checked on my condition. I was glad when morning came.

During the day I started to feel better, but I stayed in the hospital several more days while more tests were done. Two weeks after discharge, I was to see the doctor again. He ordered another test on my pancreas. Several weeks later I received a call from my doctor, advising that the test on my pancreas showed elevated activity. He said I would need to be readmitted to the hospital and have intravenous feedings to give my pancreas a rest.

My brother John had died a few years earlier of cancer of the pancreas. I had been in and out of the hospital for the past several years because of pancreatitis; I guess subconsciously I was afraid I was going to die. I purchased a physicians' medical book and discovered there was a test called ERCP. I felt this test would answer my questions. When my husband came home from work, I told him I would like to talk to him after dinner. I told him I needed emotional support because I was scared. Although Edmond had three living sisters, he started to tell me about all his brothers who had died. Although I became very upset and angry, I listened but didn't say anything.

The pain was intense as I lay in my bed. I was a bit more comfortable sitting in the chair. As I was asleep in the chair, I remember having a dream in which I saw a yellow ball of light coming toward me. The nearer the light approached me, the hotter my body became; I started to perspire. I remember thinking I was going to get burnt, when I heard a voice say, "No, but you need all this heat to burn up all the guilt, anger, and resentment that's inside you." I began to feel a great sense of peace. It was such a wonderful feeling—as though a great load had been lifted from my shoulders. The light began to fade. Again the voice spoke, "Christie, don't blame Edmond for the way he is."

4

Like the Current of the River, Which Cleanses the River of Debris

So this strong force cleansed me of anger, guilt, and resentment. I felt free and at peace.

The next day I entered the hospital. I had a series of tests performed. When my doctor came to visit, I mentioned endoscopic retrograde chalangro pancreatography (ERCP). He was afraid it might bring on an acute attack of pancreatitis. The next afternoon a surgeon told me they were going to do the ERCP test the following day. During the test I was conscious; in fact, very shortly thereafter, I was given the results. It seems I was born with a small duct and small pancreas. I was discharged a few days later.

When I arrived home, I called my attorney to make an appointment because I wanted to cancel the divorce proceedings.

The following morning, while I was working in the apartment, something told me to look inside the pockets of Edmond's jacket. My suspicions were confirmed—I found a handgun. I drove out to our place in the country and put the gun in a box of goods that we were taking to our place up north. When Edmond came home from work, he began

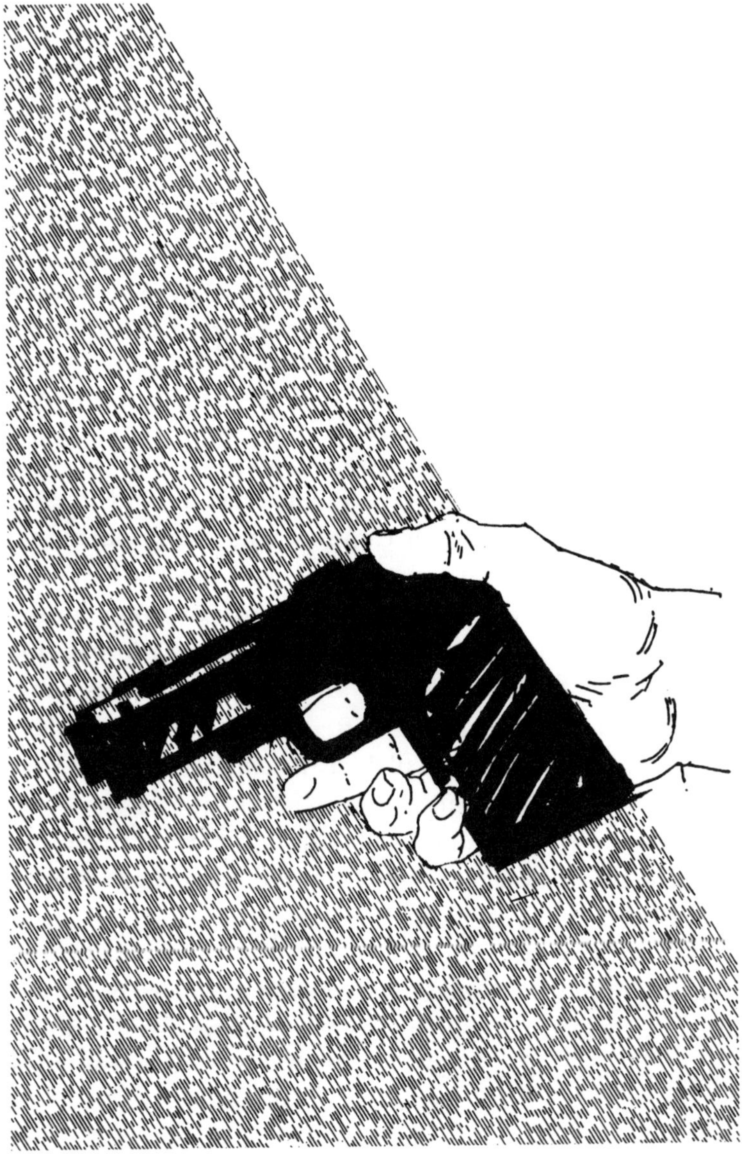

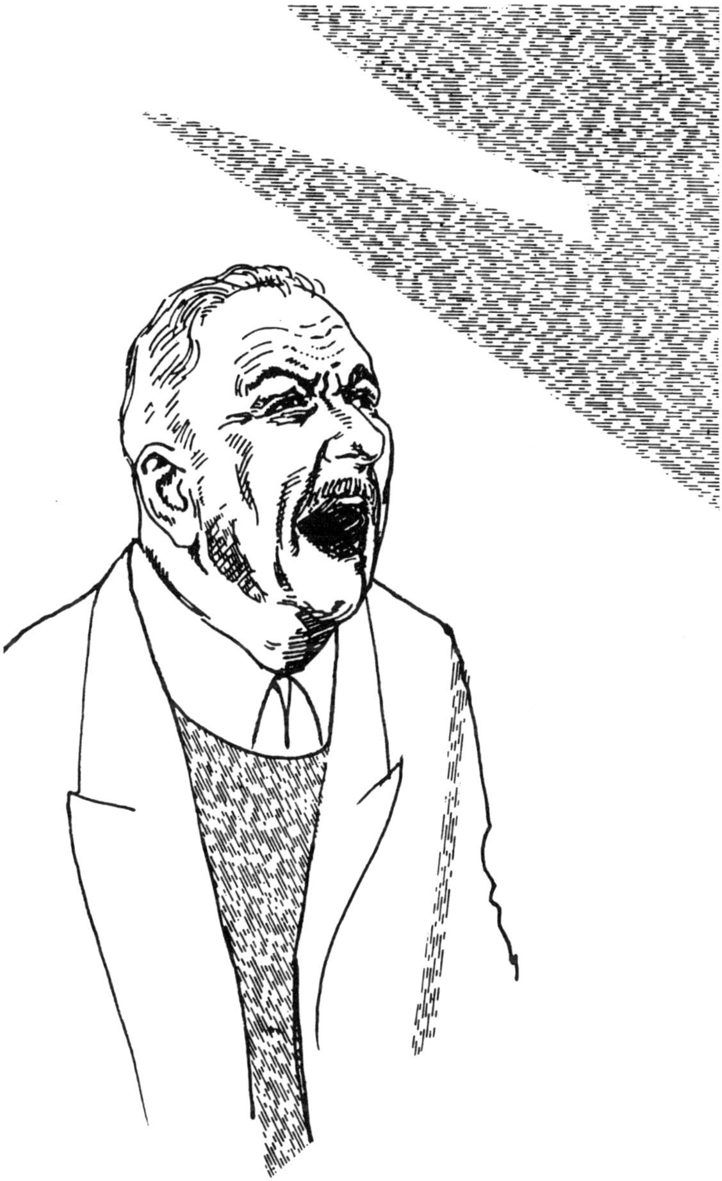

searching around the apartment. Finally, he looked up and said, "Someone broke into the apartment."

"Oh, I didn't find anything missing," I replied.

He said, "The gun is gone."

I confessed to finding the gun in his jacket pocket and taking it to the police station. He became extremely angry, started screaming, and continued to scream all night. I was afraid someone would report all the noise. He said he wanted his son to have the gun. I told him he had had many chances in the past to give his son the gun and he had not done so. A couple of weeks later, his son telephoned to say he was coming down to visit. I went to retrieve the gun and hide it in a drawer in my bedroom.

After his son arrived—and while we were eating breakfast—I retrieved the gun from the drawer and placed it between Edmond and his son. "Your dad wants you to have this gun. I don't want it in this house. Your dad has threatened suicide many times. He told me he would hold me responsible if he killed himself."

5

Like Ripples on the Surface of the River, So Were the Disturbances in My Life

By April of 1984, the relationship between Edmond and me had deteriorated to such an extent that I thought of returning to my attorney. But first there was one more thing I could try. I thought Edmond would be more at ease talking to a priest.

The first appointment involved a meeting between the priest and me, which was fine with me. The next meeting was between Edmond and the priest. The third time, both of us were present. The priest began literally to interrogate me; he asked why I was so selfish as to take Edmond away from all his friends. He continued in this manner for some time, then finally asked me why I didn't say something. I told him it wouldn't do any good as he had obviously formed an opinion about me. I began crying and ran out of the room. I was under the impression that a counselor was supposed to be objective and refrain from taking sides. I never returned.

When we reached home, I asked Edmond why he had allowed the priest to speak to me that way. He didn't answer but later told me the priest had been transferred. I decided to go back to the attorney, but this time Edmond started a countersuit. His attorney contacted my attorney and asked if

I would agree to seeing a counselor with Edmond. I answered affirmatively, so he made the necessary arrangements.

When we met with the female counselor, I explained to her that I needed emotional support, which I was not receiving from my marriage. She attempted to communicate this to Edmond, but he didn't seem to comprehend. She began role playing, but whenever she asked Edmond a question he didn't like, he would accuse both of us of making fun of him and would walk out of the session. Finally I continued seeing her alone.

In May of 1984, Edmond began to complain of back problems and took a leave of absence from work. Several weeks later he confessed that he had retired from work because, while he was doing some inspections, he simply got completely lost. At that point I think he realized that he was no longer able to meet the responsibilities required on his job.

In August of 1984, we decided to move to our place up north, as we both enjoyed the country. The scenery was beautiful, and my health actually seemed to improve for a while. I decided to work at the nursing home in the village where we lived. Still I couldn't understand my husband's behavior.

6

Like a Turbulence in the River, So My Life Seemed in a Turmoil

We were unable to sell our place in the country, so we decided to leave it. The real estate agent who handled the sale told us what his commission would be. When the place was rented, Edmond insisted on giving the agent an extra six hundred dollars beyond the agreed-upon contract rate. A few days later, I asked Edmond for some money to buy groceries. He asked if five dollars would be enough. I became furious. "I'm leaving," I said, "but before I go, I am going to the bank and withdraw six hundred dollars, which is the exact amount you gave the rental agent as a tip." He began screaming and said I needn't come back; in fact, the house would be locked. "Fine," I replied.

It was late before I took off. I was scheduled to have a session with the counselor, so I telephoned to tell her I wouldn't be able to keep my appointment. She wanted to know where I was going. I told her I would let her know when I got there. I was very upset. I began sobbing and told her I had no idea where I would go. The only thing I knew was that I needed to get away and to try to find some solutions to my problems.

After driving about fifty-six miles from home, I decided

to spend the night at a motel. The next morning I drove farther up north and I saw a motel in the country where you could prepare your own meals. I decided to stop there, as it was centrally located. I thought I would take several short trips and explore the beautiful country. There were lakes a few miles away as well as Mackinac Bridge to the Upper Peninsula; also, the Canadian border was not very far away. The people in the area were very helpful in giving me directions to interesting and unusual places. I was feeling much better, more relaxed. My thoughts became clearer, and I was better able to cope with my problems.

When I returned home, my husband was very quiet. He wanted me to see how he had cleaned the old house that we used for storage. I didn't say a thing. He had gotten rid of some wood we had stored. He had bunched things together where I had sorted and filed things; and he had piled them up in a corner. It definitely made "more room," but it certainly was a mess! It was frustrating cleaning up the mess, but I realized his heart was in the right place.

Edmond had rapid mood swings, and it was very difficult to comprehend him. It was hard for me to switch back and forth—to see him as an adult, but increasingly becoming more and more dependent like a small child. We had difficulty in communicating; he just seemed to be disoriented most of the time.

One day Edmond was driving the garden tractor and ran out of gas. He came in the house and asked if I would help him put gas in the tractor. I told him there was some in the pole barn. He seemed confused as to what I meant or what he was to do without supervision. I felt it was very important for Edmond to do as much for himself as he could, and he was happier when he was able to do something by himself. It was very difficult for me to watch him lose his many talents, but I realized it must have been more difficult for him. It upset me until I learned to look as his behavior more objectively and, above all, not to take life so seriously. However, it took a great deal of effort over a long period of time before I was able to do this.

One day he decided to fix the thermostat, which controlled heat to our furnace. It was January of 1985 and bitter cold. He had taken it apart, but he didn't have the slightest clue as to how to reassemble it. Throughout the night I had to keep turning the furnace on and off at intervals to keep us from freezing.

The next morning I telephoned a furnace repairman; he agreed to install a new thermostat before noon. I told Edmond if he ever attempted to "repair" the thermostat again, I would make arrangements to place him in a nursing home.

Later that winter we had quite a snowstorm, and by morning there was at least a six-to-eight inch accumulation. Edmond decided to take the garden tractor and scrape the snow from the driveway. He pushed all the snow into the center of the street, and plowed past our lot until he got to the neighbors' driveway. I knew I had to clear the center of the road so cars could get through. As I entered the pole barn where the tractor was kept, there was Edmond; he had taken the tractor apart. It took me a long time to shovel the snow so cars could pass through as usual. I drove to the store where he had purchased the tractor; they were very nice and sent someone to reassemble the machine for us.

February 5, 1983, is a date I will never forget. I received a call from the bank. My husband had overdrawn his checking account. I had received previous notices from the bank when he had forgotten to sign his name or the name of the person who was to receive the check. Although this had gone on for at least three years, he still insisted on having his own checking account, and I was forced to assume responsibility for paying

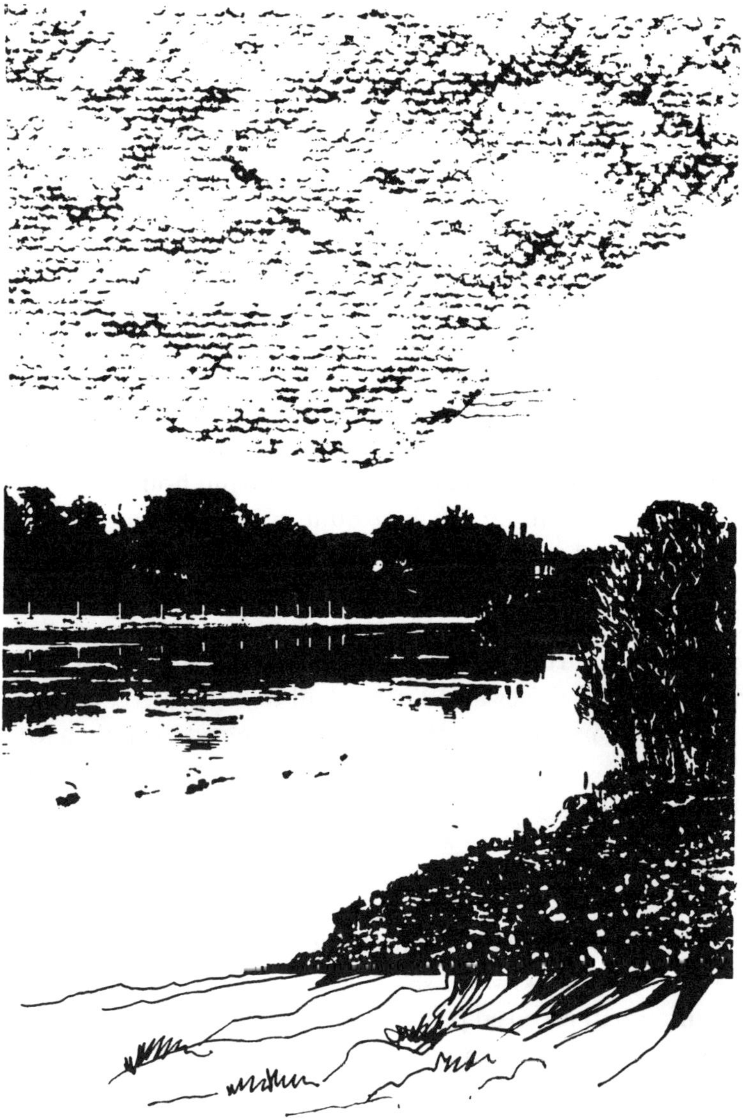

the bills from my checking account. It was not always easy keeping errors to a minimum.

Sometimes I felt as though I were on a tightrope, trying to keep my balance. Then again I saw the situation as a river I had to cross, with stones on the bottom. I saw the shore on the other side. I felt some day I would stand on that shore and my journey through these circumstances would be over. I would have new challenges to meet.

The following fall (September 1984) we decided to drive up into Canada to see the fall colors. We had always enjoyed this trip in the past, and I thought physically and emotionally I was up to handling my husband's erratic and strange behavior. In fact, I thought it would be beneficial for both of us. After crossing the Canadian border, I spotted a restaurant and a gas station. I stopped to fill the car with gas, and we had an enjoyable meal at the restaurant. Then I wanted to stop at a particular shopping mall, and as I approached the entrance to the mall parking lot, Edmond demanded I stop the car and park right there. I ignored his request; I wanted to park as close as possible to the mall entrance. As I continued to drive farther into the lot, Edmond opened the car door and got out. After some time, I finally coaxed him back into the car.

I finished shopping and we traveled farther into Canada. On our way back, I drove along Lake Superior. It's a very beautiful drive; there are many small bodies of land that look similar to tiny islands in the lake. I wanted to take pictures, so I would get out of the car and walk along the shore. Edmond became very upset and began screaming, saying there was someone out there to get me. It didn't take long before I just gave up the idea of taking any more pictures.

On our way into Canada, I had had to make many detours due to all the construction going on. It was even more difficult driving back home. As if that weren't enough, Edmond wanted to eat at the same restaurant where we'd stopped for gas upon entering Canada. I couldn't remember where it was. He got very angry and insisted he wanted to eat there. I kept driving until I was on the bridge that connects Canada with the United States. As I was crossing the bridge, Edmond opened the door; I prayed he would just stay in the car. The door closed. I drove on. Edmond was still ranting about wanting to eat, so I stopped at the first restaurant after crossing the bridge. Then and there I decided I would never take a trip alone with Edmond again.

After we returned home, I realized his behavior was so irrational that it would be extremely dangerous for him to continue to drive. I contacted the appropriate local officials, explaining the situation to them. They in turn contacted Lansing.

My husband received a summons in October to appear in Grayling to have his case reviewed. When he met with the representative, he couldn't comprehend any of the questions asked of him. Finally, the representative told my husband that it would be necessary for him to surrender his driver's license. Edmond complied. However, when he returned home, he somehow found an older driver's license and was under the impression that the older driver's license would work just as well.

7

As the Flow of a River Nears Flood Stage, So the Problems Were Overwhelming Me

Because it was increasingly more difficult to understand my husband's behavior, I decided to have his doctor make an appointment with a neurologist. The neurologist, Dr. Jeffrey C. Shephard, first saw Edmond on March 1, 1985, for his initial evaluation. He diagnosed Edmond as having a dementing illness superimposed on some suspicious personality traits. The CAT scan and electroencephalogram tests were normal. Numerous laboratory studies were also performed.

After the CAT scan, Edmond began screaming and running around the room. He said the doctors were trying to scramble his brain. It was quite a while before I was able to settle him down and take him home. A few days later, we returned for the results to his tests. When we met with the neurologist, he asked me to step outside in the hall with him. Edmond stood up and started screaming at us. He insisted we weren't going to talk about him behind his back.

The doctor later telephoned me at work to tell me that Edmond had Alzheimer's disease. At the time, I was caring for a patient at a nursing home who was suffering with Alzheimer's. The patient wasn't responding to his wife; he

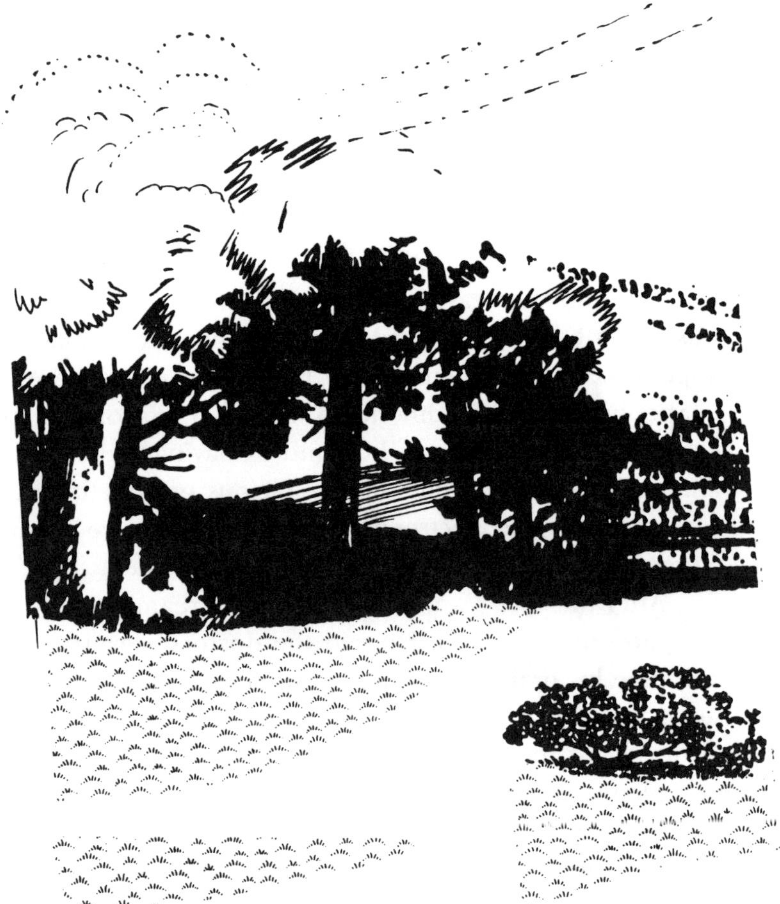

screamed night and day, and was totally helpless. A month later he died, and I felt very depressed.

I became very scared, wondering how I would be able to care for my husband. I suppose my imagination was working overtime. I felt I was in over my head and I wouldn't be able to cope with the situation. Edmond's son offered very little support, and I was told by Edmond's grandson that "the wife should resume total responsibility for this."

Later that week, we decided to go to a restaurant. I gave the waitress my order. Edmond just sat there. Finally, he asked the waitress if she would order his food. I remember feeling angry and jealous, because he didn't ask for my help, but later I realized it was probably easier for him to ask a stranger for help than someone who knew him well.

One day in May 1986, when I came home from work, Edmond told me that the sheriff had been to our home because the neighbors had tried breaking into it. A few days passed, and as I returned from work, Edmond informed me once again the sheriff had visited our home again. I decided to go to the Sheriff's Department to find out what this was all about. The sheriff informed me that my husband had aimed a gun at our neighbor. There were two rifles in the house that my husband had formerly used for hunting. I telephoned his son and told him that his dad had threatened the neighbors with a gun and asked would he please come down to pick up the guns. When his son arrived, he asked his father if he kept a loaded gun in the house. Edmond replied that he didn't. However, the gun was loaded, with one of the bullets missing. Edmond was very unhappy when his son took the guns away. He said now he wouldn't be able to go squirrel hunting; we'd better give his guns back.

One day, as we were driving down a highway near some woods, Edmond pointed to a trail coming out of the woods. He indicated a spot where, he said, an Indian had shown him the way out when he had gotten lost, even though I am sure Edmond had never seen these particular woods prior to that day. I loved this northern country where we lived. We took many pleasant trips exploring the beautiful scenery in the surrounding areas.

On auto trips, my husband was usually pretty good when it came to giving directions, but I discovered as time passed on, this was no longer the case. One day while I was driving through a town in Canada, my husband told me he knew a shortcut. I followed his directions, but we ended up in no-man's land. Finally, I asked directions at a house nearby, but we had gone a good sixty miles out of our way.

I was relieved that my husband no longer had his license to drive, even though he was not at all pleased about this. I had to do all the driving, and he would get furious when I didn't follow his directions. It became increasingly difficult to convince him that we were indeed driving in the right direction.

By summer 1986, I seemed to have more and more responsibilities. Edmond seemed to need more supervision. Many times he would get up in the middle of the night and wander around. I decided to quit my job because I felt it was no longer safe to leave my husband alone. I decided to meet with Dr. Shephard to discuss the increasing changes in my husband's personality. He was very supportive, and just being able to talk to someone who understood my situation helped immensely.

At that point in time, my husband still liked to do small jobs, but he just never remembered to put his tools away. I spent a considerable amount of time picking up and looking after his tools. If I wasn't able to find a particular tool he was asking for, he would accuse the neighbors of coming over and stealing his tools.

One day, as I was cleaning the refrigerator, I had placed

all the contents on the kitchen table. I was having difficulty with the freezer door inside the refrigerator. I couldn't fix the spring, which kept the freezer door in place. Edmond came into the kitchen and decided he could fix things. When the spring didn't go into its place, he became furious. He jerked the refrigerator door back so hard it nearly knocked over the kitchen table (now piled with food). I managed to catch the table before it fell, but a full bottle of cranberry juice landed on the carpet. Edmond had always been able to fix things and he thought he still could.

One day in the summer of 1987, two small, undernourished kittens came to our home. Edmond appeared very taken with them and wanted them to stay. I told him they weren't trained for a litter box. "Oh, yes, they are," he said. He took our cat's litter box outside and showed me how they were using it. I couldn't see how I could take care of two more kittens, but, for the first time, Edmond actually seemed to take an interest in something other than himself. He still retained some knowledge of building, so I suggested he build a house for the cats. I gathered all the material and hand tools I thought he would need.

Edmond became very interested in the project and commenced planning its construction. He had some very good ideas. The cat refuge had a loft inside, large enough for a cat to sleep on. He carpeted the loft and floor of the house. He used scraps that were left over from an addition that we had built on our house. He used heavy wood paneling for the roof. I obtained a piece of thick plastic, cut just the right size, for a window in the back. The doors were equipped with hinges, leaving them free to be opened and closed. There were fasteners to keep the door closed if necessary. He even built a roof over the door. The vinyl on the roof wasn't snug enough to fit, and this caused the house to get wet inside whenever it rained. To remedy this I bought a heavy piece of linoleum to cover the roof. It matched the paneling on the outside walls. The cat residence was large enough to accommodate all three cats. They watched Edmond while he was working; and, when he sat in a chair to rest, they would take turns lying on his lap. It was their way of expressing appreciation for the gift.

As time went on (by now November 1987), I noted that whenever I tried to explain something to Edmond, he would often ask me questions. He didn't seem to understand what I was talking about, and I would become very irate. I would become frustrated and finally say, "Just forget it." One night, after I went to bed, I had the following dream: I saw a human brain covered with a network of fine wires that didn't connect. The next morning I got out my copy of *A Guide to Alzheimer's Disease*, by Barry Rusberg, M.D. I read that certain chemicals did not make connections and therefore these messages were not received. That is why comprehension is difficult for the patient. This information helped me to adjust to Edmond's condition.

8

The River Seemed Like a Whirlpool as My Difficulties Increased Tremendously

By November of 1987, Edmond had begun wandering around at night, and I was becoming physically and mentally exhausted. I told Edmond that I needed to get away. He did not take this well at all. I told him my sister, Louise, would come and be with him while I was away. He wouldn't agree to this arrangement. As a final option, I told him either she came to stay, or he would have to go into a nursing home. It was then that he agreed to my sister's visit, and I went to a motel in Grayling. I would telephone my sister from the motel to be sure she wasn't having any problems. I stayed a week. I had taken books and knitting with me, but mainly, I spent my time resting and going out for meals.

I certainly appreciated having such a wonderful, supportive sister during this difficult time. I prayed that God would give me strength, courage, and wisdom to face whatever challenges I had yet to encounter. But it was a long time before I became adjusted to the changes in my husband's personality. His frequent mood swings made it necessary to be constantly on guard. I had witnessed an adult acting like a spoiled child and becoming more and more dependent on me. I needed and longed for an adult for a husband—not a child. I was

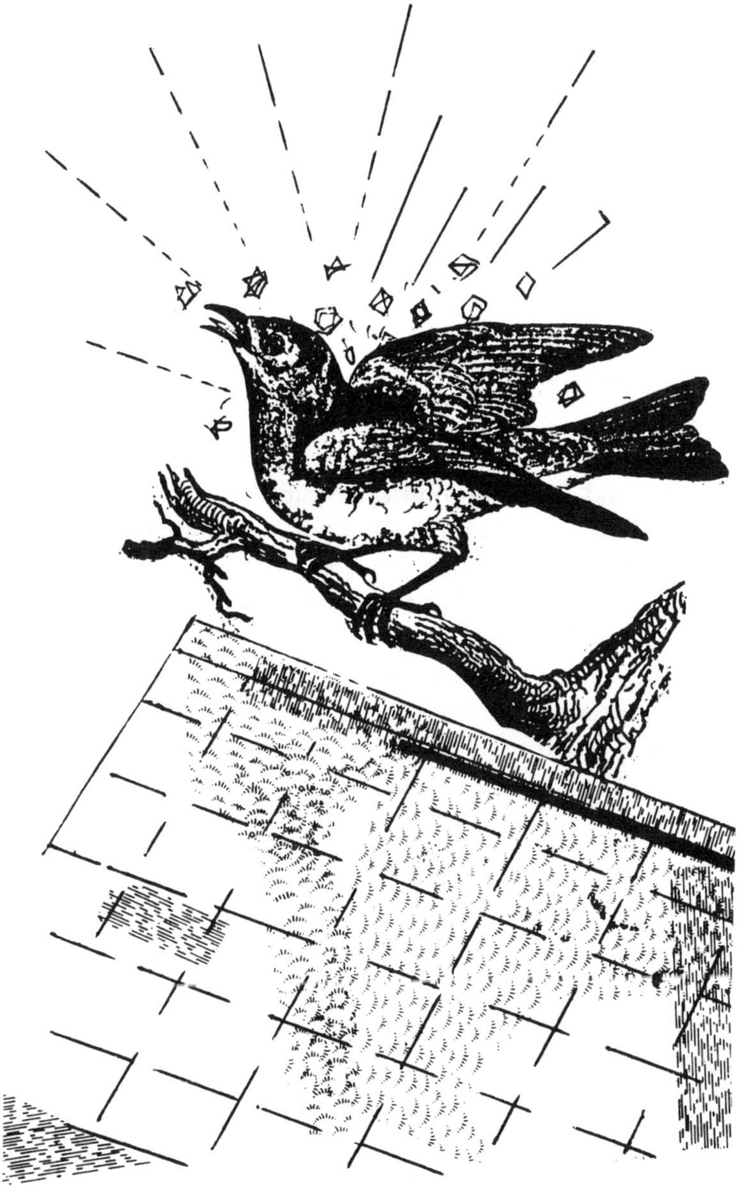

finally able to come to terms with the changing situation by continually lowering my expectations. As a result, the atmosphere became calmer and Edmond appeared to be more relaxed. It seemed my prayers were being answered.

I received plenty of help from my dreams, and I was fortunate enough to recall them in detail. I kept a record of them, and by reviewing them over and over I was able to deal with the effects Alzheimer's had on Edmond. The dreams also helped a great deal in lowering my expectations of my "new husband."

A dear friend of mine was knowledgeable in interpreting dreams; in fact, later she taught me how to interpret my dreams myself. She told me dreams were given to us in symbols, so no one else can steal our thoughts; each person has his or her own symbols.

Whenever I had a difficult day, I seemed to be compensated by having very beautiful dreams. One night I dreamt I saw a bird the size of a chicken perched on a roof. It appeared to be covered with beautiful jewels that sparkled and glowed. A child was sitting by the bird. I remember wanting to get a closer look. Suddenly, a hand reached out and helped me to my feet. I was told the bird would return in six months. (This meant there would be changes in my life every six months.)

Other nights I would see a beautiful rainbow or beautiful sunset—their beauty ineffable. Other dreams consisted of beautiful flowers, kittens, deer, squirrels, and trees. I learned to appreciate the beauty that God has given us. I learned to enjoy nature and to communicate and be in harmony with it. Life had become more meaningful, and I felt I had a more intimate relationship with nature. Gradually, I was able to view my husband's condition more objectively, without becoming overly sensitive or emotionally upset by his criticism and paranoia.

By the spring of 1988, my husband's mind had regressed

to the point at which he was behaving more and more like a small child. I felt some of his anger and frustrations might be due to fear, as it must be very scary being constantly confused, not being able to function or communicate in the usual way, to begin certain projects and, after all these years, not be able to remember how to finish them—to wonder what is happening to you.

One day when we were leaving a restaurant, Edmond stopped at the restroom. When he came out, he told the waitress someone had tried to beat him up in the bathroom. She said she would speak to the manager about it. I followed her and told her that he was my husband and that he had Alzheimer's. I never knew how he would act or what he would say when we went out to eat, but he enjoyed going out so much I hoped people would accept him.

Edmond had other health problems, too, congestive heart failure and diabetes. He refused to follow his diet, so the doctor started him on insulin injections. He wouldn't enter the hospital so he could be regulated on the insulin injections. He was afraid he would die if he went to the hospital, just as his brothers had died when they went into the hospital. So the doctor decided that I would have to start him on the injections and regulate him at home. I was instructed where to purchase the equipment and how to use it. I dreaded assuming this responsibility at first, but I realized there was nothing else to do as long as Edmond wouldn't stick to his diet.

9

Like the Gentle Flowing of the Current on Its Course in the River . . . So My Life Seemed to Flow More Peacefully

I realized that God knew me better than I knew myself. I knew God loved me very much, and there was probably some very good reason why I was to experience all this with Edmond, but it took time before I reached the point at which I began to love myself more and let God guide my life. Habits are difficult to change. Gradually, by late summer 1988, my life seemed to run more smoothly and have a deeper meaning; I felt at peace with myself. Now, instead of blaming others for my problems, I would look deep within myself to see how I could change. Thus, my attitude changed. I no longer felt sorry for myself and sorry about my present circumstances. I began to understand myself as I really was and to try to change what I didn't like. Each night and day, I would pray to be cleansed of any anger, resentment, or negative feelings. I prayed that God would help me become a more understanding and compassionate person. Thus, I was gradually able to rid myself of negative feelings and attitudes.

As I learned to love myself more, and to feel at peace, I became more loving toward others. Although my circumstances were the same, by changing my feelings and attitude,

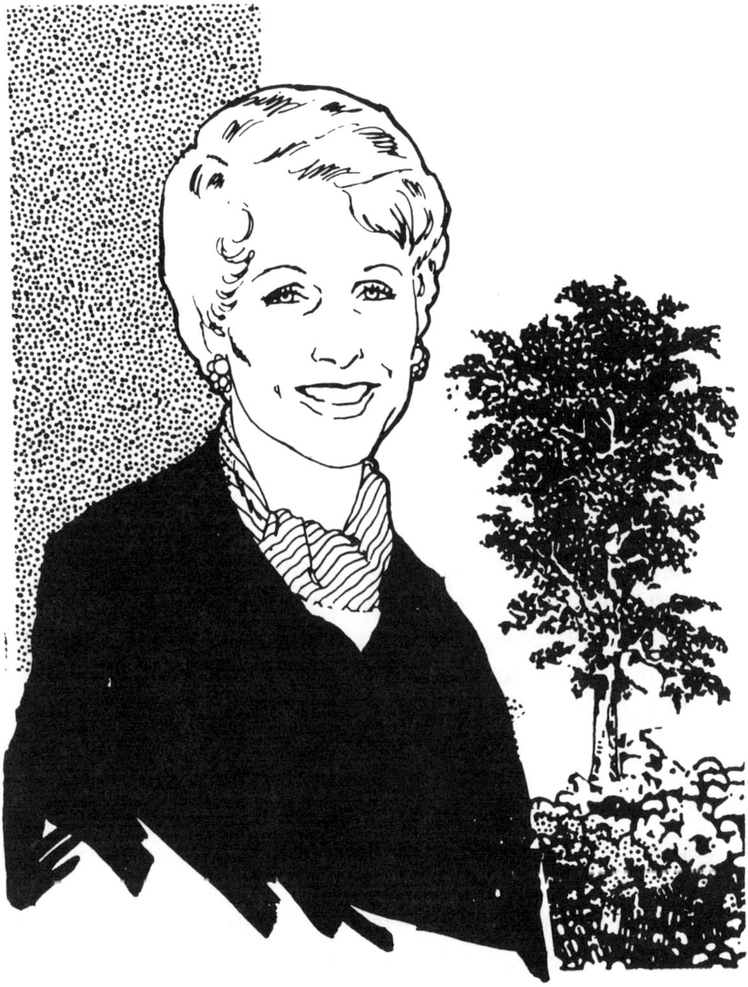

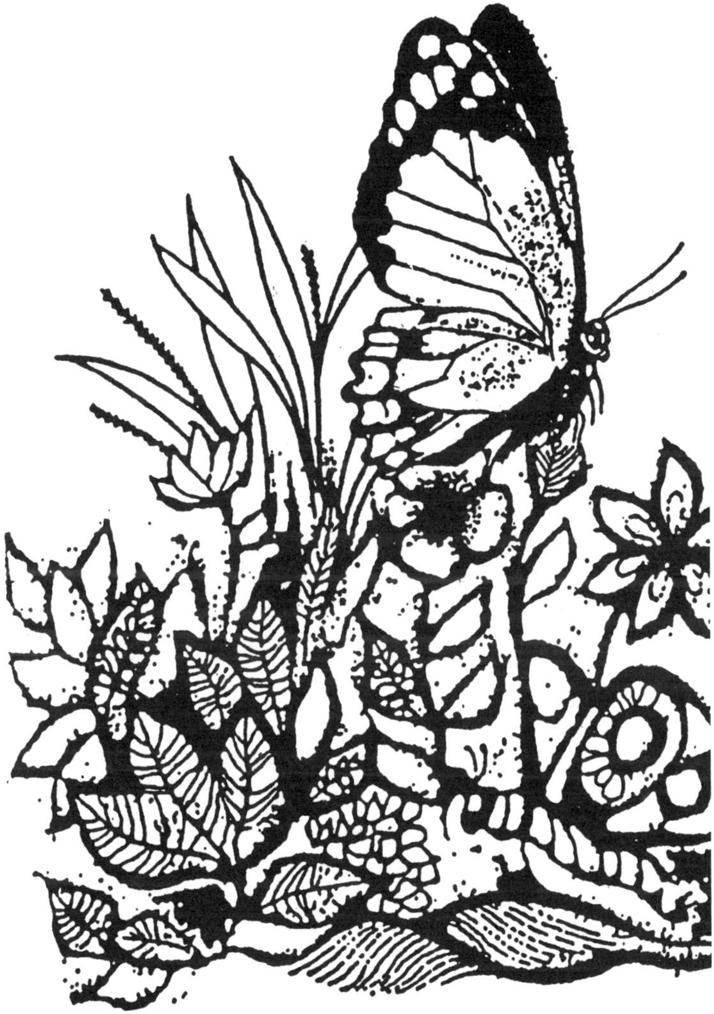

I found that the situation appeared easier to manage. I felt my life was moving forward in a more positive direction—even Edmond seemed to be more relaxed at times.

In the summer I spent most of my time outdoors. I love begonias, so I fixed a spot next to one corner of the house, which was shaded, and I terraced it up three tiers. It became quite a showplace and was greatly admired by everyone. I spent time admiring and closely observing nature, carefully examining the leaves on different trees and plants. I watched the birds and animals that came into the yard, as I spent many pleasant hours working in my vegetable garden. It was quite a challenge because of the change in the weather and the limited time I could spend there due to my other responsibilities. Our last frost was in June, giving us only a short growing season. I had to grow vegetables adapted to a cooler climate, learning this through trial and error.

10

The Changing Currents of the River Were Like the Changing Events in My Life

Living in a confused state, not being able to remember anything, and not being able to communicate very well became increasingly frustrating for Edmond. At times I felt guilty because I lacked more patience; as life became more difficult, not being able to express my feelings seriously affected my health. Edmond didn't seem to want to go anywhere but out to eat. He refused to have anyone else stay with him, and he resented any visitors. Things would have been easier if I had been able to get away once in a while.

By summer 1988, my husband refused to have any visitors in our home. As much as I wanted to join a support group, I couldn't leave him alone. I made an appointment to see Dr. Shephard as I was still having difficulty adjusting to the many deepening changes in my husband's personality. Just being able to talk to someone who understood my circumstances was very helpful and lessened the stress.

Because Edmond would not cooperate with his doctor about his health problems, the doctor again suggested placing him in the hospital. But again, Edmond refused. The doctor told me that because of Edmond's mental status and his inability to make decisions, he would need a legal guardian. I

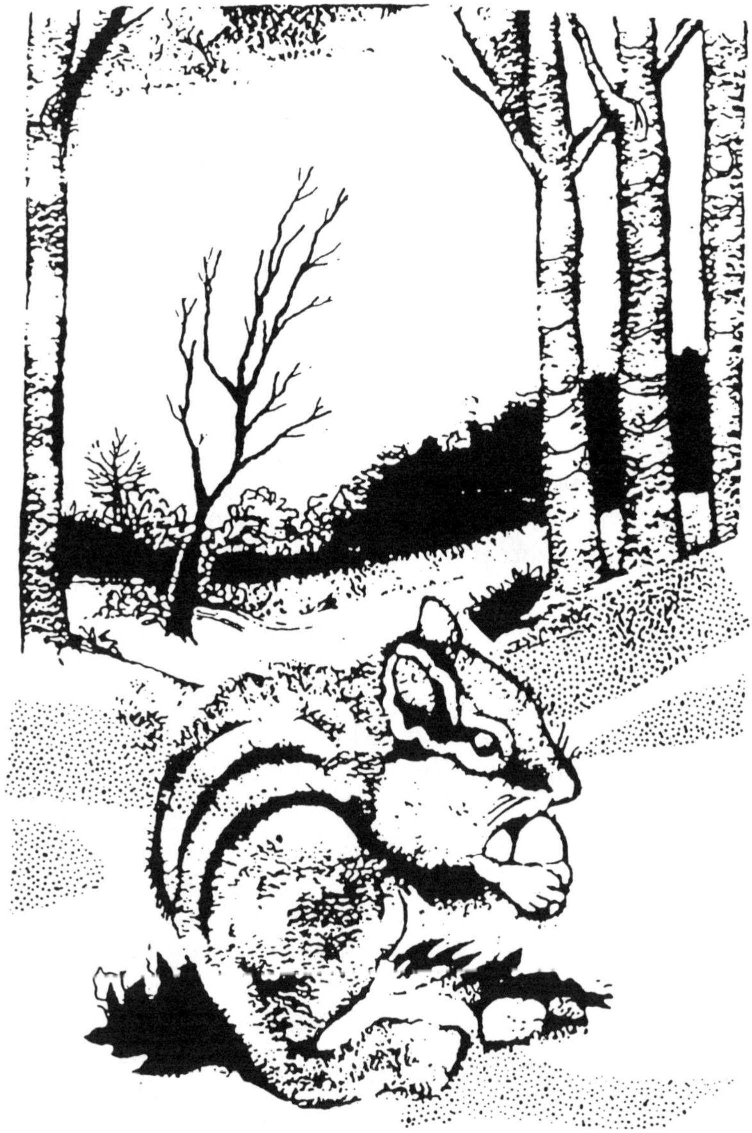

never realized when I made the commitment to become his legal guardian the demanding effort it would entail. I hired the same Grayling attorney I had used for small matters in the past. I had had very little experience dealing with attorneys. In court I was to give a full account of all assets that were in my name and Edmond's, also both our incomes, and any joint property. The hearing was scheduled for July 20, 1990, and a notice was sent to his son.

At the hearing, testimony was given regarding Edmond's health and mental deterioration during the past few years due to Alzheimer's disease. I had been managing his affairs for his benefit. However, as he now refused necessary medical treatment, medications, and diet recommendations as prescribed by his doctor, he was placed in my care.

A written testimony was given by Edmond's doctor, along with results of a neurological consultation obtained in May 1990. It stated that Edmond had dementia and was unable to make decisions in his own best interests. Also, he might need immediate placement in foster care or in a nursing home as I was not able to control him. However, Edmond refused to go either to foster care or to a nursing home, so I continued to care for him in our home. Also included in a medical report during the hearing was a statement of how Edmond would use an assortment of tools trying to repair electrical wiring, although he had no formal training or qualification. He repeatedly extinguished the lights. I was afraid he would be electrocuted. During the hearing he was asked if he wanted me to take responsibility for his financial and business affairs. He said yes, as I had been doing this all along and he stated he didn't want anyone else to do this.

Because of his refusal to have anyone else in the house to help me care for him, my own health began to suffer. Three different doctors advised me to place my husband in a nursing home; a priest even suggested I use force. But I just couldn't do it—even though I had repeated bouts of pneumonia. I finally became so exhausted caring for Edmond without any help from anyone, I told him one day he would have to go into a nursing home so that I could get some rest. He said he wouldn't go unless his son was there.

I made arrangements for him to enter Bortz Nursing Home in Rose City, which was sixteen miles away. I had inspected the home. I liked the way it was managed and the number of activities they had available for the residents.

On May 1, 1991, Edmond's son and grandson, John, came over. My husband wanted to talk to his son privately, so I went into the other room. When I reentered the room, his son told me Edmond wanted him to see about funeral arrangements. I then showed him a letter from the funeral director, who was Edmond's cousin. It contained information pertaining to the details of funeral arrangements I had made for Edmond. His son told me he had made the same funeral arrangements for his mother when she died. He explained this to his father. Edmond was satisfied with this arrangement.

We then proceeded to take my husband to the nursing home. His son was pleased with the general operations at Bortz. We both stayed until Edmond had quietly settled in.

Most people assume employees at their social services department will be helpful, warm, and friendly. Think again. All I can say is I hope you have better luck communicating than I did. I filled out all of those lengthy applications to see when Edmond would be able to qualify for Medicaid, because up until this time we had been paying cash for Edmond's stay at the nursing home. When I met with one of the workers, I was told to provide the following information: a list of assets, which included all savings accounts, checking accounts, CD savings, stocks, also the amounts we each received from Social Security, or any other payments from pensions, annuities, land contracts, trust funds, or payments from property sold; also any payments received from any other investments if they were joint or personally owned by myself.

Even though certain CDs and savings were in my name only, they were considered joint because we were living together. Even a paid-up insurance policy of mine, which was paid up before I even married Edmond, was taken into account. I had taken the money from the policy and invested it in stock. Because of inflation, and the cost of funeral expenses, I had decided I needed the extra income the stock would provide. I felt it was unfair to call this "joint."

The social worker questioned the amount of stock and the benefits that I was receiving, as though I weren't giving a true account. I gave him the address where he could write for verification. After one and one-half months went by, I returned to the Department of Social Services to inquire why I hadn't heard about my application for Edmond. My social worker said he had been too busy to work on my application. I then contacted a lady from Agency on Aging, a long-term-care ombudsman, who gives assistance to people having difficulties. She agreed to meet with my attorney. She discussed with us what steps were necessary before my husband could qualify for Medicaid. She suggested we go back to Social Services to find out why I still had not heard from them. My attorney telephoned for an appointment. When we arrived at the DSS office, my attorney inquired again as to why we had not heard from them. The social worker said he had been too busy. It seemed that on that particular day he had turned my case over to another worker. He then called that worker into his office. My attorney looked over the copy of my application and then handed it to me. When I checked the application, I noticed there was a discrepancy: one of the saving accounts I had submitted to the DSS office had been omitted. When I noted this, she handed me a copy of the application that I filed. (I just wasn't getting anywhere with these guys.)

I decided to visit another DSS office, one that was located in the same county Edmond's nursing home was in; and I made an appointment to see a social worker there. The social worker wanted the person in charge of the office to go over my case with him.

I gave him all my receipts, bank statements, and other important documents that he requested. After a couple of weeks, they told me my case was so complicated that they would have to start at the beginning.

Instead of taking the amount of savings and other assets we had at the time my husband was admitted into the nursing home, they took the amount of assets we had when they started their evaluation, which made quite a difference. I didn't notice the error at the time, which was my fault, but I felt something wasn't right. I was told I could keep 50 percent of the savings and assets. It was two years later before I was able to clear up the mistakes, with the help of Congressman Dave Camp and Jan Osborn, LTC ombudsman from another organization. The whole situation caused me considerable stress, which ultimately affected my health.

Conclusion

Edmond seemed to be adjusting to his new home. I made frequent visits, and we always went out to eat. Sometimes we would go for rides in the country, as he liked to see the wild turkeys and deer. As time progressed, he seemed more at peace with himself and was enjoying socializing with the staff and residents. I believe he was happier because he felt he didn't have to compete with the exigencies of our daily life.

There were many activities available for the residents at Bortz Nursing Home, in Rose City. The atmosphere there was very homey, and the residents were treated with respect. J. R. Marchal, the director of the home, spends time daily visiting with residents. As he makes his rounds, he lets all the patients know that if they ever have any problems, he is available.

I told the activity director that Edmond had held positions where he was in charge. Also, that he loved music, dancing, and playing the violin. The director suggested that I bring his violin to the nursing home. She allowed him to lead a group in music with his violin. He also took part in a project they had at Christmastime. Edmond told the activity director that he had been a security guard at one time. So when they had a party, she had Edmond check the people coming into the party. He also helped make the nativity scene. He attended their church services every Sunday and communion services on Tuesday.

The nursing home also provided outside activities for

those able to attend. One time it was a boat ride down the river. There was dancing; my husband had always been a great dancer and he really enjoyed himself. He was quite excited when he told me about the good times he had. Other times, they held outdoor picnics, which he really enjoyed. He seemed to feel comfortable at Bortz and was much calmer and kinder whenever I visited.

Although Edmond has had Alzheimer's for at least eighteen years, he still can feed himself and has control of his bowels and bladder. He needs help with shaving and dressing, and usually spends much of his time in a wheelchair. I had to discontinue taking him out to eat due to his weakness; it became too difficult for me to handle him. When I visit Edmond, he keeps telling me he wants to go home. I keep telling him I cannot take care of him, as it takes two people just to transfer him from his wheelchair to his bed and vice versa. But it upsets me when he keeps wanting to come home. At these times I feel guilty and depressed. It is very difficult to carry on a conversation when I mention certain incidents or ask if his son called. He tells me he saw him on TV or saw the incidents on TV.

Sometimes Edmond knows me and sometimes he doesn't. He gets along well with his roommate, and he takes an active part in the activities at the nursing home. He is calmer and more relaxed, and there is a slower deterioration of his mental condition.

It was quite an adjustment for me after I placed Edmond at Bortz Nursing Home. I had surgery for breast cancer, followed by radiation, which exhausted me; stress had affected my health more than I realized.

It was quite a change to be around people I could communicate with after spending so much time with a person so mentally unbalanced and diminished, but as time went on, it was easier to adjust to other people.

In winter of 1993, a pheasant came to my home. I observed it needed sand to be able to digest its food. I placed a pan of sand by his food. After that he would always come at a certain time each day to eat. The pheasant was enjoyed by everyone in our neighborhood. He loved chasing cars; he'd run up and down the street chasing them. One day he didn't come to eat. I looked for him down the street, but I didn't see him, so I crossed the street and found him lying dead on his side by the curb. I buried him in the back of our vacant lot. My neighbor missed the pheasant and asked me what had happened to him. I told her he had been killed by a car. She told me he had roosted in her evergreen tree every night. She said it made her winter more enjoyable because of him.

In August of 1994, my sister, Louise, and our friend, Vera, came for a visit. We picked Edmond up at Bortz to take him to dinner. Later we brought him home to see the cats. Red, a neighbor, came over to see Edmond. Edmond became exceedingly angry. It appeared he didn't want to share his visitors with anyone else.

One day in November of 1994 was the last time I took Edmond out to brunch in West Branch. A young man from Florida had to help me get him back into the car, so I realized I wouldn't be able to take Edmond out by myself anymore.

Bortz had a mobile dental unit so that the residents were able to receive any dental care they needed. Also, a medical doctor made calls at the Home, so Edmond didn't need to leave for his medical care.

In February 1995, I received a call from Bortz that my husband was ill and not responding. The doctor had ordered X rays and lab work, and Edmond was given intravenous feedings. He had pneumonia. I was ill myself at that time, so I wasn't able to see him for two days. On the day I visited Edmond, he was still having intravenous feedings, but he was able to respond to me. I sat and held his hand while he slept.

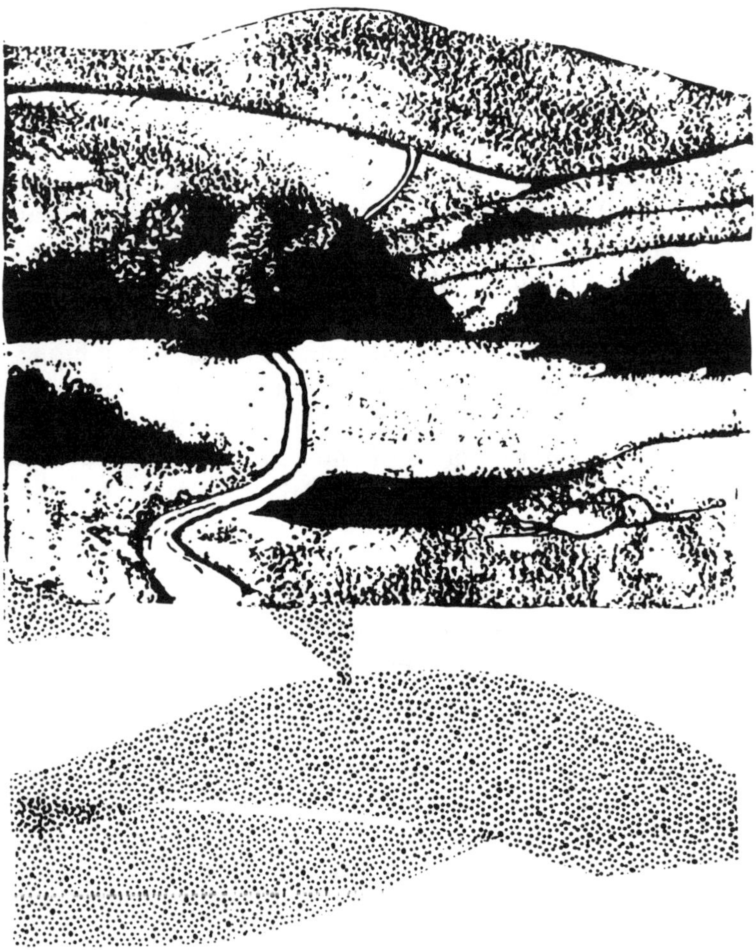

The next day when I visited him, I was surprised to see him coming down the hall in his wheelchair. He had pulled out his IV and insisted on getting in his wheelchair. As I continued to visit him each day, he seemed to improve quite rapidly. But he had lost a great deal of weight. He now required side rails on his bed, and because of his weakness, they didn't want him to try to get out of bed by himself.

I realized Edmond's health had continued to slowly deteriorate. I realized I had to make further adjustments in my life as circumstances demanded. But I was now able to make them in a more positive manner than I had for many years.

Like the peaceful flow of the river, so my life became more peaceful and enjoyable as I developed a closer harmony with the beauty of nature. I enjoy walking by the river that is near my home. The scenery there is so beautiful and peaceful. It is wonderful to watch the water flowing down the river.

Emil or Edmond died mar 22 1998